**CARING ABOUT
YOUR WHOLE BODY**

THE VEGAN

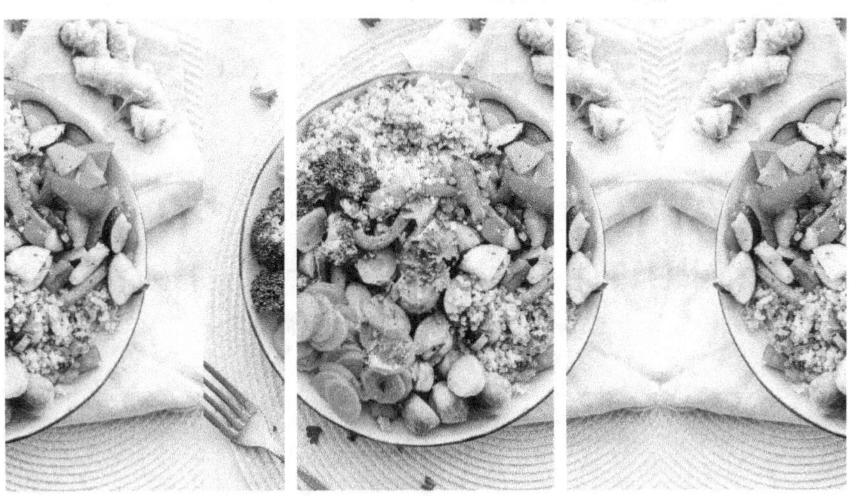

WEIGHT-LOSS PLAN

Health Writers

MEDICAL DISCLAIMER

This book is created and published for informational purposes only. It is not intended to be a substitute for professional medical advice.

Always seek the guidance of your doctor or other qualified health professional with any questions you may have regarding your health or a medical condition. Never disregard the advice of a medical professional, or delay in seeking it.

TABLE OF CONTENTS

MEAL PLANNING TECHNIQUES

MEAL PLANNING GUIDELINES

MEAL-PLANNING ADVICE

1. PICK A MEAL-PLANNING METHOD THAT SUITS YOU.

2. MAKE A GROCERY LIST OF PANTRY AND REFRIGERATOR ESSENTIALS.

3. SET UP YOUR KITCHEN WITH EVERYTHING YOU'LL NEED.

4. SET ASIDE A DAY TO PLAN AND SHOP.

5. ASSESS YOUR WEEK AND MAKE FOOD PREPARATIONS AS NECESSARY.

6. READ THE LABELS ON THE FOOD

ON A VEGAN DIET, HOW LONG DOES IT TAKE TO LOSE WEIGHT?

WEIGHT LOSS SPEED IS AFFECTED BY SEVERAL FACTORS

FACTOR 1: ARE YOU CHANGING YOUR DIET?

FACTOR 2: WHAT IS THE TOTAL AMOUNT OF WEIGHT THAT YOU NEED TO LOSE?

FACTOR 3: DO YOU HAVE A PARTICULAR BODY TYPE?

FACTOR 4: DO YOU FOLLOW A HEALTHY VEGAN DIET?

<u>CONCLUSION</u>

INTRODUCTION

Have you been a vegan for some time but haven't lost any weight? Read on for some possible reasons why you're having trouble losing weight as a vegan!

Many individuals believe that losing weight on a vegan diet is straightforward. They believe that turning vegan will cause them to lose weight regardless of what they consume, as long as animal products are avoided. This is an extremely common misunderstanding.

This myth that "veganism equals weight loss" is incorrect, as many vegans discover. Indeed, if you are not following a healthy vegan diet, it is rather easy to gain weight. Chips, cookies, cakes, "cheese," and other processed foods are readily available to vegans. For everything, there is a vegan option!

This is excellent for the animals and the environment (and cheat days!), but if you want to lose weight on a vegan diet, you need to consume the RIGHT foods the majority of the time.

WHAT TO KNOW ABOUT VEGAN ALTERNATIVES

Beyond Burgers, vegan butter, and vegan cheese are just a few of the vegan options available. It's so tasty, but it's also so bad for you! Treat yourself now and then, but eating this type of food daily will make losing weight much more difficult.

Vegan cheese recipes may be found online, and they're a terrific alternative to store-bought processed cheese. There are plenty of delectable vegan burger recipes available as well!

Make sure you always have healthy food on hand so that when you're hungry, you don't reach for anything quick and processed!

Menus that don't contain any meat

During veganuary, jackfruit appears to be a popular option. The ripe fruit has a sweet flavor, indicating its close relationship to the fig, whilst the unripe fruit is salty and has a fleshy texture. Because of its fleshiness, it's a great alternative to pulled pork in curries and burgers.

The problem is that, if you're looking for protein, jackfruit is nutritionally useless. It's largely carbs with very little protein. It is not a good meat substitute.

Other plant-based protein sources are also inferior to animal protein sources in terms of quality. Proteins are made up of amino acids, which are the building blocks of all our cells and hormones. On the other hand, most plants lack sufficient quantities of all essential amino acids.

Plant-based protein sources are typically deficient in at least one of the nine essential amino acids, which the human body requires but cannot synthesize and must obtain from food. Vegans must either carefully balance their proteins so that they complement one another, or supplement their diet with other sources.

Meat, eggs, and dairy products, on the other hand, are termed "complete" foods since they provide all nine required amino acids.

If your protein diet consisted completely of lentils and beans, you would get some but not all of them." Vegan burgers often include beans, but they aren't the only source of protein. Soy is a fantastic foodstuff since it contains a lot of good protein. My go-to protein would be that.

Another difference in quality between animal and plant-based diets is the amount of iron they contain. While many vegetables are high in iron, such as whole grains, lentils, and spinach, it is not always the greatest variety. Haem iron is found in animals, while non-haem iron is found in plants. The body doesn't absorb non-haem as effectively as haem. Iron deficiency is an issue, especially for women who require more iron throughout their menstrual cycle.

In a meta-analysis of iron deficiency studies in vegetarians, vegans, and omnivores, vegans (especially women) were found to be the most at risk. According to one study, 25% of vegans, compared to 3% of vegetarians and 0% of omnivores, had extremely low blood iron levels. Vegans are particularly affected by even slight iron deficiency (30 per cent, compared to 21 per cent of vegetarians and 0 per cent of omnivores).

Food pairing is crucial

If you're going to stay a vegan for the long haul, some foods contain compounds that help other foods absorb chemicals more quickly. When we take a non-haem iron source, for example, we can boost our absorption by taking vitamin C. When cooking with lentils, Rossi recommends starting with a tomato foundation that is high in vitamin C.

It's also important to think about what goes into vegan fast food to make it as satisfying as meat alternatives. For example, a vegan KFC burger in the United Kingdom has 2.91g of salt, compared to 2.02g for their fillet burger and 1.97g for their Zinger burger. In addition, the vegan burger contains more sugar, carbs, and protein.

OIL-FREE EATING MAKES A DIFFERENCE

The health implications of oils have sparked a lot of discussions. Some study suggests that particular oils are beneficial to your health, while other research suggests that all oil use is harmful to your health. This can be perplexing, so if you're undecided about whether or not to consume oil, I strongly advise you to conduct as much research as possible and make your own decision.

After doing some research, I've chosen to stop using oils because I believe they provide no health benefits and may harm my body. Oil is just fat that has been taken from entire foods and has a high caloric density. A tablespoon of oil has about 120 calories in it, which your body doesn't require! It's simply a waste of calories, and more calories mean weight growth.

Eating an olive rather than simply the fat is taken out of it is significantly healthier. You'll get more nutritious value from the whole olive. Coconut oil is a similar case. Coconut oil has recently received a lot of attention as a health food; however, studies show that it elevates dangerous LDL cholesterol levels. It's just like any other oil when it comes to toxicity.

How can oils be removed from your body?
In many recipes, I've discovered that the oil isn't required because it's merely used to aid in the cooking process. For stove-top sautéing, you can substitute vegetable broth or water. If the flavor complements what you're preparing, you can even use soy sauce or tamari.

However, eliminating oil from baking recipes will radically alter the texture and perhaps destroy the recipe. Applesauce or mashed bananas, or even liquid sweetener, can be used in its place. Look for vegan baking recipes that don't use any oil. They do exist, and they're fantastic!

Oil-free eating is becoming increasingly popular, particularly among vegans. Is it necessary to eliminate oil from your diet, as some plant-based doctors recommend, to achieve optimal health? The answer, as with any nutrition question, is often subjective.

Oil-Free Diets' Health Advantages

If endothelial function research is restricted, isn't there more compelling evidence for avoiding oil in the diet?

A few other studies have found that eliminating oil from one's diet has heart-health benefits. People with heart disease (who had already had a heart attack) were put on a 100% whole food, plant-based diet, according to one study that is frequently quoted (including the elimination of oil). Further cardiac incidents were shown to be extremely rare in those who adhered to this dietary program.

This is an intriguing study, and while I do not believe it should be dismissed, it is crucial to consider all of the information while conducting research.

Oil-free diets are thought to help with weight loss as well. Because oil contains a great number of calories in a little amount of space, the calories from the oil can quickly stack up without physically filling a person up. While consuming more food to consume fewer calories is one way to lose weight, it is far from the only way.

There's also a distinction to be made between being physically fulfilled and feeling satisfied. Fats and oils might make you feel fuller after a meal, which means you're less likely to eat again soon.

Finally, there is a distinction to be made between taking a small amount of oil and drowning a meal in oil. While the word "moderation" may not be popular, it is an important one to remember. Adding 1 tsp or 1 tbsp of oil to a meal is not the same as eating anything that has been deep-fried or coated with a lot of oil.

THE POWER OF PORTION SIZE CONTROL

Many people have told me that portion control is unnecessary when eating a whole-foods plant-based diet. Some argue that if you eliminate all manufactured foods from your vegan diet, you can consume a limitless amount of the good stuff and still lose weight.

You're unlikely to lose weight if you eat a pot of potatoes every day or eat a lot of peanut butter. Avocados, potatoes, rice, all-natural peanut butter, and all-natural peanut butter are all good for you. Hopefully, you get the picture. However, if you consistently consume these foods, you will find it difficult to reduce weight.

If you wish to use peanut butter in your oatmeal, use one tablespoon, but don't consume a few spoonfuls straight from the jar. If you're attempting to reduce weight, I'd also suggest only eating half an avocado at a time. Avocados are delicious, but they can pack up to 300 calories depending on their size.

Eat a lot of fruit and lots of green vegetables, however, there are some healthful whole foods that you shouldn't eat in excess. So, if you're eating well but not losing weight, check your portion sizes!

You might also try cutting down on good fats, but don't go too far! Because every person's body is different, there is no one-size-fits-all approach to eating.

If you've tried everything else on this list and are still having trouble losing weight, you may need to experiment with your portion sizes.

The most common cause of weight gain is overeating.

You will acquire weight if you consume more calories each day than you expend.

Excessive calorie intake is promoted by mindless eating, frequent snacking, and consuming calorie-dense, nutrient-poor foods.

If you struggle with overeating, visit a licensed nutritionist.

Paying attention to hunger and fullness cues while eating mindfully are some basic techniques used to avoid overeating.

It is not true that following a vegan diet will allow you to eat as much as you want while remaining thin and healthy. Indeed, this perspective may be the reason you're still binge eating, believing that the sky is the limit when it comes to portion sizes.

Overeating can be avoided in two ways

1. Recognize the high-risk scenarios in your life.

Each individual's situation is unique. You may overeat in public or in private; you may overeat during a mid-afternoon slump, or you may be unable to manage late-night desires despite having eaten dinner. Whatever the case may be, you are likely to overeat at a particular moment or in a specific setting. It's straightforward to establish techniques to manage these situations after you've determined which periods are problematic for you. Put these techniques into action when you're at your most vulnerable. If late-night snacking is a problem for you, you may discover that you need to eat your mid-afternoon snack close to the time you're going out to dinner so you don't overeat in a restaurant, or that you need to set a cut-off time for stopping to eat in the evening. Whatever your high-risk overeating period is, the objective is to control it.

2. Learn to recognise whether you're hungry or full

Many of us consume so much food or consume it so frequently (or both) that we can't recall the last time we were hungry. I'm not advocating that you starve yourself (in fact, this is a Food Effect guideline), but if you can't recognise true hunger, it's also tough to know when you're full. Many of us may merely feel stuffed or uncomfortable at this time. If this is the case, pay attention to when you begin to feel full and pleased.

It takes at least 10–20 minutes for the stomach to register true fullness, and even longer for the food you consume to reach the end of your intestine, where more satiety hormones are generated, so it's usually a mouthful or two before the actual full feeling. Before deciding on seconds, give it some time. Between mouthfuls, set your cutlery down and chew slowly. This will assist you to measure how your body is feeling so that you don't eat on autopilot like a machine – and, as I previously stated, eating slowly will guarantee that your brain detects when you've had enough food before it's too late.

MEAL PLANNING TECHNIQUES

Many people understand what they should eat to lose weight on a vegan diet, but many struggles to follow through. I'm aware that there are occasions when I'm feeling particularly lazy and don't feel like preparing a nutritious meal.

Meal preparation comes into play here. Meal planning and prepping may be helpful if you have trouble staying on track.

Meal Planning Guidelines

I'd recommend looking for healthy vegan recipes online or in a cookbook and choosing a couple to consume throughout the week. Check the portion sizes and alter the ingredient amounts as needed to ensure you have enough food for the week.

It may be good for you to select meals that share some of the same components so that you do not have to purchase as many groceries or waste the ones you do purchase. If you choose a half-onion recipe, for example, choose another half-onion recipe so that you can use the entire onion.

Once you have all of your ingredients, make all of your dishes on the same day and store them in the refrigerator in containers. Then you'll have a ready-to-eat vegan breakfast, lunch, and dinner each day!

You'll be far less likely to reach for something unhealthy during mealtimes as a result of this.

Meal-planning advice

1. Pick a meal-planning method that suits you.
Various people have different ideas about what meal planning should look like.

Some people prepare a grocery list based on the meals they'll cook and eat over the week.

Other others prepare all of their meals for the week ahead of time and portion them out using meal prep containers, so they only have to cook a few times during the week.

Others have a mix of both!

Select the meal-planning method that best suits your needs. Remember, the point is to plan your meals for the week; you can prep as much or as little as you wish ahead of time.

2. Make a grocery list of pantry and refrigerator essentials.

Meal planning is made easier and less frightening by keeping your cupboard and fridge stocked with essential supplies.

This ensures that you eat well and prepare nutritious meals at home. The initial expenditure may appear big if you are working with restricted ingredients. Recipe selection and grocery list creation will be lot easier once you have these essential components.

3. Set up your kitchen with everything you'll need.

Make sure you're on the right track! When you don't have the right tools, it's difficult to prepare and preserve meals. Knives and pans, as well as storage bags and containers, are all examples of proper kitchen equipment.

4. Set aside a day to plan and shop.

Due to time constraints, I normally plan and shop on Sunday, although planning on Saturday and shopping on Sunday is easier for me. Choose a day that is most convenient for you! Keep these days consistent to help you organize your days and meals.

Of course, there will be occasions when you need to purchase or plan on a different day, but remaining consistent will help you make meal planning a weekly habit.

5. Assess your week and make food preparations as necessary.

It's time to get serious about meal planning now that you have the necessary tools, essential ingredients, and a designated planning/shopping day.

Consider the coming week: early morning meetings that necessitate grab-and-go breakfasts, a Friday lunch with coworkers, evening soccer practice with your kids, and so on. Any circumstance or incident that will affect your cooking time or ability should be mentioned.

Stick to your strategy, but be willing to change it if necessary.

After all of that hard work, it's understandable that you want to keep to your schedule, but there may be days when unexpected events occur or you simply don't have the stamina to complete your task. That's fine; just have a backup plan in case something goes wrong.

6. READ THE LABELS ON THE FOOD

It's important to remember that just because something is labelled "vegan" doesn't mean it's healthy. Pay attention to the ingredient list and the calorie count per serving. Don't be deceived by serving sizes that appear to be small to make the calories appear lower.

Make certain there are no oils or extra sugar in the ingredients. Sugar is frequently listed on ingredient lists under a different term that you may not recognize as sugar, so learn more about sugar's alternate names.

You've probably heard it before, but if you can't pronounce it and/or have never heard of it, you shouldn't eat it. Not at all, especially if you're trying to reduce weight!

Looking for a label that says 'Suitable for Vegans' or a 'Certified Vegan' emblem is the simplest way to tell if a product is vegan. Scanning the 'Allergen Information' is another simple technique. If a product contains dairy, eggs, or seafood, the allergy ingredients list will mention so. Check for the Green Dot to see if it's vegetarian.

Make your way to the 'Ingredients List' if the first two methods don't provide enough certainty. You can use this tool to look for non-vegan components and chemicals. But what should you be looking for specifically? Animal products and derivatives can be found in even the most seemingly benign products, such as biscuits and cosmetics.

Veganism is more likely if the product is vegetarian and does not appear to include any animal byproducts.

Another thing to remember is that if a product says it may include' an animal ingredient but doesn't say so on the label, it's usually safe to eat.

This is because firms must do so to avoid being sued if a customer has an allergic reaction to an ingredient that was mistakenly included in the product during manufacturing.

Don't let this deter you from purchasing such items; it doesn't indicate that animal products have been flying around the factory where they're made, and it doesn't mean that you're not supporting a product that contains animal products by purchasing it. That is crucial.

If you're new to eating a healthy plant-based diet, you might be having trouble figuring out which things you can and can't put in your cart. Nutrition labels and ingredient lists can be perplexing, particularly if you're not sure what you're searching for. Of course, the majority of the foods you'll buy on a whole food plant-based diet (fruits, vegetables, dry whole grains, and legumes) will not require you to read ingredient lists or labels. However, for some products, such as whole-grain bread, plant-based milk, and condiments and sauces, you'll need to know how to read labels. This will assist you in making well-informed selections about what to buy and what to return to the store.

Finally, you may believe that calories are the most significant (or even the only) factor to consider when reading a nutrition label, but this isn't totally true: 300 calories isn't 300 calories if the pack contains three servings. If you consume twice or treble the portion size, what you believe is a low-calorie lunch could end up costing you 600, or even 900 calories. Make sure a serving size (and how many additional portions you eat) fits into your daily caloric allowance by doing some quick math.

ON A VEGAN DIET, HOW LONG DOES IT TAKE TO LOSE WEIGHT?

Veganism is an excellent strategy to shed pounds. Vegans, in comparison to meat-eaters and even other vegetarians, have a lower average BMI (body mass index). But, if you're a vegan, how long does it take to shed pounds?

Vegans have lost anything from 5.6 pounds in 18 weeks to 7.5 per cent of their body weight in six months, according to research. The speed with which you lose weight as a vegan is determined by several things, including the diet you're transitioning from and the amount of weight you need to drop.

Each pound of fat contains around 3,500 calories (source). To lose 10 pounds of fat, you'll need to expend around 35,000 calories.

Vegans consume 600 calories per day less on average than meat-eaters, according to one study. So, if we divide 35,000 calories by 600 calories each day, a vegan may lose 10 pounds in around 58 days (two months).

On a vegan diet, you could lose 63 pounds in a year at that same average rate of calorie burning (if you have that much excess fat to lose). That isn't a certainty, though. It differs in practice.

Indeed, vegans have been observed to lose weight at a substantially slower rate in some studies. A vegan diet for 18 weeks (just over 4 months) resulted in an average weight loss of 5.6 pounds, according to this study. That does not appear to be a particularly quick weight loss. Also, keep in mind that weight loss with keto is usually quicker. (Vegan, on the other hand, is healthier and lasts longer.)

Overweight persons who followed a vegan diet for six months dropped an average of 7.5 per cent of their body weight, according to one study. (For example, if you were 200 pounds, you would lose 15 pounds in six months.) That has a greater impact.

However, I am aware of some vegans who did not lose weight. As a result, it differs greatly.

Weight Loss Speed is Affected by Several Factors

Here are four major influences on how rapidly you lose weight as a vegan:

Factor 1: Are you changing your diet?

It's possible that a vegan diet won't speed things up too much if your diet was previously health-conscious. If you've been eating fast food and processed garbage, switching vegan may help you lose weight much more quickly and dramatically.

Factor 2: What is the total amount of weight that you need to lose?

You'll probably drop more pounds per month if you have more body fat to lose. Weight loss may be slower if you're only slightly overweight.

Weight reduction tends to slow down as your body reaches its target weight. Your body is resisting your efforts to reduce all of your body fat! (However, I'll give you some advice on how to lose "the last 10 pounds" further down.)

Factor 3: Do you have a particular body type?

Another factor is genetics. Ectomorphs are naturally thin, whereas endomorphs are overweight.

You may be an endomorph if you've always been a little overweight. As an endomorph, you can still lose weight—it simply won't be as easy as it is for others.

Factor 4: Do you follow a healthy vegan diet?

The meals you consume have a significant impact on your overall health. Vegan foods can still be harmful and simple to consume too much.

To sum up, if you need to lose a lot of weight and have been eating a bad diet, being vegan for a few months could help you shed 10 pounds or more. Others will see a slower rate of weight loss. Veganism isn't a quick fix.

If you aren't seeing the weight reduction results you want, there are several things you may do to improve your diet.

Overall, try to be patient and make just the necessary adjustments. It's not uncommon for folks to devote a year or two to achieve a significant and long-term physique transformation. You, too, can arrive. It simply needs the correct strategies, which must be implemented consistently over time.

CONCLUSION

While converting to a vegan diet can lead to weight loss, it is not guaranteed. It all depends on what you ate before you went vegan and what you consume now. You will almost certainly not lose weight if you started eating processed junk food and then switched to vegan junk food. A healthy vegan diet that is based on plants, on the other hand, can help you lose weight and keep it off.

Veganism can aid weight loss. However, before making major dietary changes, it's usually a good idea to see your doctor or a dietician. You should talk about where you'll receive key nutrients like protein and B vitamins.

Your doctor may also prescribe alternative weight-loss strategies, such as keeping a food diary or following a regular exercise programme.

www.ingramcontent.com/pod-product-compliance
Lightning Source LLC
Chambersburg PA
CBHW070229260726
48658CB00006BA/2233